I Have Epilepsy, so Let's Talk . . .

I Have Epilepsy, so Let's Talk . . .

Stephanie Gallet

Copyright © 2018 by Stephanie Gallet.

Library of Congress Control Number: 2018910746
ISBN: Hardcover 978-1-9845-5216-7
       Softcover 978-1-9845-5218-1
       eBook   978-1-9845-5217-4

All rights reserved. No part of this book may be reproduced or transmitted in any form or by any means, electronic or mechanical, including photocopying, recording, or by any information storage and retrieval system, without permission in writing from the copyright owner.

Scripture quotations marked NIV are taken from the Holy Bible, New International Version®. NIV®. Copyright © 1973, 1978, 1984 by International Bible Society. Used by permission of Zondervan. All rights reserved. [Biblica]

Scripture quotations marked NKJV are taken from the New King James Version. Copyright © 1982 by Thomas Nelson, Inc. Used by permission. All rights reserved.

Scripture quotations marked NLT are taken from the Holy Bible, New Living Translation, copyright © 1996, 2004, 2007. Used by permission of Tyndale House Publishers, Inc. Carol Stream, Illinois 60188. All rights reserved. Website

Scripture quotations marked KJV are from the Holy Bible, King James Version (Authorized Version). First published in 1611. Quoted from the KJV Classic Reference Bible, Copyright © 1983 by The Zondervan Corporation.

Any people depicted in stock imagery provided by Getty Images are models, and such images are being used for illustrative purposes only.
Certain stock imagery © Getty Images.

Print information available on the last page.

Rev. date: 10/29/2018

To order additional copies of this book, contact:
Xlibris
1-888-795-4274
www.Xlibris.com
Orders@Xlibris.com

CONTENTS

Gratitude vii
Preface ix
Introduction xi

Chapter 1   How It All Began 1
Chapter 2   Everyday Life 3
Chapter 3   Who, What, and When 11
Chapter 4   Relationships 15
Chapter 5   Let's Work around It 19
Chapter 6   Not Another Day 21
Chapter 7   Three Life-Changing Surgeries 23
Chapter 8   A Little Humor 29
Chapter 9   Through the Eyes of Loved Ones,
             Family, and Friends 33
Chapter 10   Unconditional Love 37
Chapter 11   Where I Am Now 39
Chapter 12   Troubling Relationships 43
Chapter 13   Don't Lose Hope 65
Chapter 14   A Huge Help 67
Chapter 15   Scriptures 69

A Final Thought 71

GRATITUDE

I AM EXTREMELY GRATEFUL to my aunt Debbie Bushey. This book wouldn't have been possible without all of her care and support. I am also thankful to my husband for believing in me. I wouldn't have gotten this done if he didn't have faith in me.

PREFACE

THE REASON WHY I wrote this book is to share with you some of the struggles that come with epilepsy. Of course, all of us are different. Let's look at it like this. We may wear the same shoes, but we don't all wear the same size. We just need to walk together to know that we are not alone. This is regarding all disabilities. We can work together to overcome the obstacles that come with our disorders. We can learn from one another and look at all of it with a positive attitude.

I know that it isn't easy for any of us. I myself have had a difficult time getting to where I am today. We can do it! We cannot let this disorder or any type of illness get the best of us.

Oh yeah, one more thing that inspired me to write this book is when God brought it to my attention. So let's look at it today as a new day and live it as if it were our last. It is healthy for us to let go of the past and focus on the future. Let's just give it to God and trust that he will take care of us.

INTRODUCTION

AS YOU ARE reading this, you are probably curious of who is explaining his/her experience. If we were meeting in person, I would introduce myself like this: "Hello, nice to meet you. My name is Stephanie. I am a forty-three-year-old woman who has epilepsy."

I have had surgeries—one on the right temporal lobe and also on the left. I will explain more later. I was eighteen years old at the time of the accident. I had a seven-month-old child.

I am writing this book for those of you who want to understand, care to learn about, and be able to relate to this disability and the difficulties that come with it.

Although this book is about me and the troubles I have had, it is for you or someone you may know who suffers with epilepsy. Who knows, maybe even some doctors and nurses will learn from this. People will not know or understand what we are going through unless we explain it. The more that we share, the more they will learn.

I am definitely not a writer. I don't even read books. I am having a hard time comprehending what I read. This has been a problem all my life, but now it is much more difficult.

CHAPTER 1

How It All Began

WHEN I WAS eighteen years old, I came into some money and my first thought was to buy a car. I had a driver's license, but I had never owned a car.

Luckily, I only live a mile or two away from a dealership, so on my birthday, I put on some tennis shoes and paraded down the street with a smile on my face, thinking, *Today is the day that I am going to find the perfect car for me.* So without anyone's help or advice, I anxiously followed my plan to buy a car.

When I got to the car dealership, a gentleman approached me and asked if I would like to take one of the cars for a test drive. I didn't know why I picked the one I did. I was sure this came to mind: *Wouldn't I look good driving this?* Maybe the dealer could see how fast my heart was beating through my shirt. The one I chose was a two-door bright-red sports car.

I cared more about how the car looked and not about how it would drive. It was definitely not the right car for me. I didn't even get another person's opinion before buying it.

My struggle with epilepsy was brought on when I was in a severe car accident at the age of eighteen on April 2, 1993. I was told that after the accident, I was flown to the closest trauma center, Loma Linda University Medical Center.

My mother was called to come identify me. They did not expect I would live through the night.

I was in a coma for a week and was in the hospital for a month. This was when my seizures began.

After coming out of the coma, I had no idea what had happened. I had no memory of the accident or that I had a son who was in the car with me.

I did, however, remember my mother, father, aunt and grandparents, whom I loved dearly. This was disturbing to me. This was the beginning of my memory problem.

CHAPTER 2

Everyday Life

MANY THINGS IN our everyday life can bring on seizures. Stress has been one trigger that have brought on mine. Those of you who have epilepsy may have experienced other triggers, such as smells, good or bad. Others are the smell and taste of food.

My mother made many meals where I had to leave the room because of the smell. The smell of popcorn had always, in the past, brought on at least one seizure. Usually, a petit mal. There have been other types of food, yet I now cannot remember exactly which ones they are. However, I know I also had troubles with the smell of perfume and cologne. It had been a problem in the past to hug friends, families, or acquaintances being that they might have some type of smell on them that would bring on one of these petit mal seizures. I usually stayed away from even looking into finding the one perfume or body spray that I would be able to handle.

I am sick and tired of these so-called episodes or seizures. You have no idea of when or what happens when you have them. Sometimes, you don't even know that you did have one. I don't know about you, but they have turned my life upside down. Some of you may have had them since birth and are used to them.

Mine started when I was in a car accident with that car I had just purchased. I was in a coma for a week and in the hospital for a month.

For the first decade after my accident, my mother and I were on welfare using Medi-cal to get by. This was because I needed her to help watch over my son and me. We needed her care twenty-four hours, seven days a week. She wasn't able to work for a long time. If I didn't have the medical insurance from the county, I don't know what I would have done.

I had trouble remembering what had happened in my life the week before. I was now aware of how very important our memory is to us, in our everyday life. I often felt like a forty-three-year-old woman with the brain of a child.

Some people, including myself, do not want to remember certain occurrences from the present or the past. In my case, I don't have a choice. I just need to go with the flow and live in the moment. I have always admired people who are able to do this. I just need to get in the habit of it. My everyday challenges would be a lot less stressful for me if I do. Sounds good, huh? It would be a great weight off my back. I am sure people around me would like it if I did this. So now that I am giving this a thought, I would like to start this today. I can do this! All of us and you—if you have a hard time with something like this—can do it too.

It is all about us getting in the habit of waking up each morning and asking ourselves, What can I do to make my life better today?

Everyday Struggles

I am embarrassed to admit that I have a constant habit of dwelling about all kinds of things. People often remind me, "The past is the past." So in some ways, the memory problem is good for me. When you are disabled, there are so many things to dwell about.

Well, I am sure that many people would rather not be in a conversation with someone like me who dwells about a problem that they cannot fix.

I often share my feelings with God and pray that I will change, which I have in many ways. I am doing all that I can to get this disorder out of my life. God has guided me in the right direction, even in writing this book.

Disturbing Situation

I have had a great many times when I cannot find something, and my first thought is that somebody has it. They took it from me. Where did they put it? This might be just *a short time* after I saw the item or even had it in my hands maybe just an hour or so ago. It is so upsetting when I think that someone I know and care about, who also care about me, would take something (such as an item of jewelry or even food that I desire) from me. This makes me so angry, yet the anger fades, then other emotions take over. I would sometimes find it a day or two later. I have a habit of hiding items that I don't want to share or lose.

Since the surgery, I, of course, don't remember where I have put these items. My next thoughts are, *Why would they have taken this from me? Was it just to upset me?* After a while, I forget all about it. Sometimes forgetting can be a positive thing.

What Do You See?

Since day 1, I have been very interested in what I look like when I am having a seizure. The people around me who have seen this happen (a great many times) have explained to me what I looked like in just a few words. They may say something such as "You fall down and your body shakes externally" or "Your eyes roll back, and you sometimes drool." I have been told that I would mumble about what it is I am seeing while I am having the seizure. It is such a scary feeling. I have no idea what is going on around me. It is when I see visions of something that I have seen before but has never happened. They are like dreams that I recognize. I sometimes explain what it is I am seeing. They are more disturbing to me than the grand mal seizures. They are very intense. They are the ones that they call déjà vu seizures. That is the perfect word for them. I am not as tired when I have this type of episode. I can, after a few minutes, go back to what I was doing before I had it. These haven't bothered me half as much as the petit mal seizures. I don't believe I have ever seen anybody have a seizure in person. Oh well, I don't wish it on anyone, so I don't care if I see anyone have one.

Today is the day I got an idea of what it looked like. My best friend and I had spent a few days together, and in one of our conversations, I explained to her that I would always be curious of what it looked like. So after our little talk, she came up with an idea, showing me on the computer of other people who have had one and what it looked like. As she was showing many pictures, she would explain it something like this: "Here's what you look like when you are having one of those kinds of seizures. And that is what you look like when . . ." She did a very good job at helping me, but of course, I don't remember any of it.

Another special time that touched my heart was when my husband showed me a video of me having a seizure. By writing this book and sharing my experience with epilepsy, I am hoping that it will inspire others to share the experiences (with any kind of disability) that they have. There is so much more to our disabilities than what those around us see. So let's share our feelings and help others to learn from them.

All of us are different; however, the more we learn from one another, the better it will be. It will open up our minds and open the doors. We will have more information to look into and speak to our doctors about. Instead of just listening to what they want to do, hoping that it may be helpful that way, you will have the ability to let them know what you have learned about and you can find out if it would be beneficial to you. This is what I regret not doing before having my three surgeries. I would have had more confidence in my life-changing experiences. With the trouble with my memory, I should keep a diary of all that is going on, and this may be good even for those who have a good memory. There is nothing negative in doing this. It is only going to be positive and be helpful to the doctors. We just need to keep a pen and maybe a small notebook with us at all times. This will be a great help to us and the doctors.

Nobody but God knows what is to come in our future. We can only hope for the best and do our best to make it a positive one.

Many times over the past twenty-five years, I have gone to a great deal of doctor's appointments that did not seem to be much help to me at the time. I would go at least once a month. This was when my seizures were at their worst. Although, I don't remember those years specifically, I do know that I had petit mal seizures almost daily. I recall waking up every morning with frightening feelings—the same type of feelings I have had after having a petit mal seizure.

Some of my seizures only go on for a minute or less. I personally call these "feelings." They are also known as auras. I am not conscious of what is going on around me when they occur. An example of this is when my girlfriend and I would go out dancing when we were younger. After the accident, people around us told my friend that they thought I was drunk, but that is impossible because I don't drink alcohol. The atmosphere of carnivals and casinos and the sound of bells and rain would bring them on. The smell of certain foods, like popcorn, the smell of perfumes, the taste of some foods, and flashing lights would also bring them on.

That is why I am here for you, to share how all of it has affected my life.

Yes, I still do get a little upset even with the positive changes in my life to help me get over this disability, but as many say, I need to be patient and fight this disorder.

It is such an awkward feeling being free of seizures for this long or at least not having the memory of what it was like when I did have them. My husband has explained to me that I have had a few since my last surgery. Maybe the RNS just needs to be adjusted a bit. We will see. Time will tell. Yet I am not aware of any of the ones that I have had since the surgery about six month ago. I haven't had a doctor's appointment since then. Of course, I don't remember when my next appointment is coming up.

I am just thankful that UCLA knows what they are doing. They are the highest quality health care. I am totally secure and confident in their medical decisions to advance my health and well-being. They have put a lot into all this, and it touches my heart that they haven't given up on me and all the obstacles that I have gone through. This RNS surgery is new to all of them. But as I have told you, I am willing to do anything to live without these seizures. It would be a dream come true. I have total faith that God is leading me in the right direction. I do not want to get overanxious.

That is how important it is for people who have a disability to communicate with others who can understand what it is like.

Wouldn't This Upset You Too?

Just a few moments ago, I felt like a child again. Something happened to an important family member of mine, and I would have liked to be a part of helping to solve this problem. But as it would be for a child, I just stood back and watched others take control of the situation. I couldn't do anything about helping someone who needed my help.

I was not upset with the person who did what they were able to do. It was just my jealousy of being a person who did not have the ability to go where I want, when I want, or when I am needed. It was greatly upsetting to live this way. It was disturbing to look like you were all there on the outside but not on the inside. This quote just came to my mind: *You shouldn't judge a book by its cover.*

I am thankful I don't struggle being in jail or living on the streets. This epilepsy is torturous. I know for a fact that there is no way I would be able to survive in that type of lifestyle.

I met a woman yesterday who was having a hard time with her spinal cord injury. How annoying that might be, but as we were talking, she showed me the surgery she had. She explained to me that it hadn't been much help. A quick thought came to my mind as she said the words "I want to get a second opinion." After I asked, she told me which hospital it was that she was getting all this done at. It was the same hospital where I started. The one I told you that did nothing for me.

CHAPTER 3

Who, What, and When

*E*PILEPSY IS WHEN a seizure interrupts normal brain activity—not just a little but a lot. It is a problem that is known to affect approximately one in fifty children and one in a hundred adults. If this is true, then why don't more people talk about it? The two types of seizures that I have are known as petit mal and grand mal. Petit mal seizure (I have learned) are also known as simple partial seizures. All I know is that these seizures start with a terrible feeling in your body and mind. These do not last long. Sometimes, it is less than a minute or two, but they are extremely disturbing.

In my case, I am much more disturbed by the petit mal ones compared to the grand mal ones. This is because it is greatly upsetting when you have no control over the visions you are seeing and the way your body and mind are reacting to them.

I often ask God, "Why me? Why any of us?" There are so many of us good citizens who don't deserve this. I also think of all the many criminals who are in good health—maybe not mentally but physically. I feel for any person with a physical or mental illness.

It just disturbs me that I do not know when these seizures are about to occur.

We need to take time to investigate what comes with it. It sounds good in the beginning, but what are the consequences with the surgery? I had a magnetic device in-planted in my chest. It is known as the vagus nerve stimulator (VNS). I was to wear a magnetic bracelet around my wrist. I was to put my wrist on to my chest where the device was. This was to eliminate the seizure. However, as many of you can understand, when the seizure is about to start, you don't think externally; you are just concentrating on the visions you are seeing in your mind. And with the grand mal, when you are so overwhelmed with all that is going on, you don't have the time to think to put it to your chest.

Sorry, I Do Not Remember

As a result of the surgery of the right temporal lobe of my brain, my short-term memory has gotten extremely worse. I sometimes wake up in the morning having no idea what happened the day before. I may remember something about it if I take some time to think it over, but in this fast-paced world, I do not have much time to do that. And even when I do, I am probably going to forget about it afterward.

Therefore, I get extremely disappointed with myself and my thoughts. If I cannot remember the details of what happened the day before, then there is no chance of me remembering what has happened in my life the week before. I am now aware of how very important our memory is to us, every day of our lives.

When I look back at some of the conservations I have had with people, I have noticed that I use the word *I* an awful lot. This is not because *I* am a conceited person. It is mostly because that is all *I* can remember. There *I* go again.

I am not able to remember which team won which game or which actor was in which movie or even what the move was about. I work at a grocery store, and thank goodness for all the signs hanging from the ceiling, giving me an idea of what is where. After working at the same store for ten years, you would think I would have it down pat by now. So when someone asks me where something is, I just say, "I will help you find it."

Most of the time, since I have had the surgery on the right temporal lobe, I don't even know when I have had a seizure. This is much better than me knowing or feeling that it is about to occur. Now I don't know that I have them. People tell me when I do, and it is a total surprise to me. If I have gotten this far, then I can't give up now.

CHAPTER 4

Relationships

IN THIS CHAPTER, I am going to explain to you about the relationships that I have in my life as I struggled with epilepsy. If you have epilepsy, you may be able to relate to these situations.

I was living with my son and his father before the accident. I frequently kept in touch with my family. So when I got out of the hospital, my mother became a great help to me and my seven-month-old son. She cared for us 24-7. I could not be left alone. She had to quit her job and learn about epilepsy, just as I did. She did it with a loving heart. I had doctor's appointment once a month, that she took me to. She cooked meals for us daily. She didn't want me to cook. She was afraid that I would have a seizure. And of course, that was understandable. I'll talk more about that later. We lived on aid until the two of us could get back on our feet. We had to go to a county hospital, which wasn't very much help to me. Well, not as helpful as the hospital I go to now. All they did was change the dosage of my medicines at every visit. There is no way I could have taken care of my son on my own. I could not even take care of myself. I was in desperate need of her help. She did a great job caring for us both.

My mother made so many sacrifices. There was just one problem. She was able to give my son all he wanted and needed, whereas I could not. Now the relationship with my mother sure did have ups and downs.

It was jealousy I had for my mother who was caring for my son. The stress of this brought on more seizures, one after the other. My mother was a very special person to me. I wouldn't be here today of I didn't get all the love and care that I got from her. She loved and cared for my son. This affected my relationship with her and him. Maybe if I was in good health, my son would love me more. He was just too young to understand. I felt more like a sister, not his mother.

Now for some good relationships. I have two best girlfriends—one who has epilepsy and one who does not. Both of them have been great blessings to me.

The one who does not have epilepsy does her best to understand what I am going through. She has been there for me through thick and thin. She has been a huge help to me during the hard times that I have been through. She has stuck by me and helped me as my mother did. She is definitely what you would consider a best friend.

The other girlfriend I met after my accident, and she also has epilepsy. She lives across the United States. We met when some people put a bunch of us epileptics together to learn more about one of the medications we were taking. It was a free trip that flew me to another state, so why would I pass it up? Plus, I got paid for explaining my experience with epilepsy. We connected right away. We had a lot to talk about, and we still do. I am so thankful for telephones. It means so much to me that we keep in touch. She does know what it is like to live with this stupid disease. We have both put up with a lot. We have a great deal in common and can relate to each other and the troubles that come with epilepsy. We both have terrific husbands who care for us with unconditional love.

It is so important to have friendships. All of us with any type of disability should stay in contact and communicate with others that can relate.

The most valuable relationship for me is the one I now have with my husband. I am now a happily married woman with a job that I enjoy. My husband and my employer wanted me even with this condition. When I met my husband, my seizures were consistent. Before I met him, I would ask myself, Why would anyone want to be with a person like me? There are so many women out there who are in good health.

He had stood by me through so much since the day we met and had never complained about any of it. He had a heart of gold. I met him a decade after the accident. And this was when I was having seizures frequently. A relative recently told me that when we were dating, he went to the library to find books about epilepsy. He didn't know anything about it before this. Kind of cute, huh?

Stress is known to bring on seizures, so fortunately, I don't have to worry about that when it comes to my husband. He knows how to deal with me when I am stressed out.

Well, I do what I can with what I've got. I just know that I would not be able to have gotten this far if I didn't have all the love, care, and support that my husband gives to me daily. The first words that come out of his mouth every time I call him are "Is everything okay?"

I usually reply with "Yes, why do you ask?"

Then with a loving heart, he answers me by saying "Because if you're okay, then I'm okay." Who doesn't want to hear that?

CHAPTER 5

Let's Work around It

I DON'T KNOW about you, but I have always been in need of work while having this disability. This doesn't have anything to do with being in need of money. Yet the more money I make, the better, especially when you have hospital bills and extra expenses, like medications. I have been working since I was sixteen years old, but after the car accident, when I was having one seizure after another, I had to stay home. I was still determined to stay busy because I would rather use my brain on work instead of thinking about what television show I was going to watch next. My memory was somewhat bad in the first years; however, it was not anything like it is now.

For example, there was one job I had in the past that I would never be able to have now after the surgery (where they took part of my brain out of my head). I once applied for a job as a waitress. I had no trouble getting the job, even with the difficulty of my everyday seizures. As I look back, it was such a surprise that they accepted me with no fears of me dropping plates. I would put a pleasant smile to my face and say something like "If I remember correctly, you are the one who is craving this meal." Maybe once in a great while I was wrong, but I was lucky that most of the people tell me which one was theirs before I put the plate on the table in front of the customer I was hoping who ordered it. I always went home with a smile, especially after I received all my tips of the day.

Another occupation I had was when I got a job as a secretary from a gentleman who I had unexpectedly met. As we were casually talking, he brought up to me that he was in need of someone to do all his paperwork and data entry he didn't have time to do. After he asked me if I was looking for a job, I shared with him the medical complications I was having with my disorder. After explaining the health problems, he said, "Don't worry. We will work around that." He was such a wonderful inspiration to my life. He did not complain about any of the seizures. He just taught me what I needed to know and had total faith in me to do the work that he taught me.

I have had a good number of jobs since day 1. I have always enjoyed working, and I have never been fired from any of them. All of my coworkers have been supportive and caring. I am currently working at a grocery store, bagging groceries and putting items that weren't purchased back where they belong. After ten years, it is still my favorite job. I still have some trouble remembering where some of the items belong. Thank goodness they have signs on each isle to let you know what is where everything belongs.

All my jobs have been a gift from God to me. I don't know what I would have done if I didn't have them. I would definitely have been bored in this life.

I have no regrets having this surgery on my right temporal lobe if this is what it takes to reduce or put this disability to an end. I cannot let these seizures control me. I just need to do what it takes and give it my all.

Always remember that God is the doctor, the church is the hospital, and we are the patients. He will take care of us.

CHAPTER 6

Not Another Day

SPEAKING OF MY life, I tried to take mine twice. Now that I look back with the chance of being seizure-free, I realized how stupid that was to do to myself and those around me, especially to my family, friends, and the doctors that have put so much into helping me get better with all that I have gone through with them. The first attempt to end my life was after one of my brain surgeries—the one where they take a piece the size of a quarter out of my brain to help control the episodes I was having.

I have a tremendous problem with everyday stress in my life. I may be smiling on the outside, yet I am frowning on the inside. We all have some type of stress in our lives. It is how each of us deal with it that matters. Those of us who have a disorder or disability have a lot more to overcome. Life is difficult as it is, so why do we need any more discomfort in it? It is the stress in my life that is my enemy. You may be thinking, *Don't we all have stress?* Stress is known to bring on seizures, so it makes my life even more stressful, which brings on more seizures.

All of us who are suffering are in need of more support and care than the average person. Because if we don't have it, we may want to give up. But tomorrow is a new day, and it may be a good one. So let's not lose hope.

Who am I to talk? But look how far I have come. We can all do this one step at a time and grow from our experiences.

CHAPTER 7

Three Life-Changing Surgeries

I HAD A surgery where I had the VNS implanted into my chest. This was the one that the doctors at UCLA had talked to me about on the day of my first visit with them. VNS stands for vagus nerve stimulator. I had never heard of this before, have you? Well, it was more popular now than the day I had learned about it.

When the doctor brought this surgery to my attention (after many years of waiting for these words to come out of a doctor's mouth), he asked me if I was interested in having this done. I anxiously said, "Of course, let's do it! The sooner, the better." I didn't give it a second thought. I was very excited about this.

Now that I look back at it, I should have researched it, found others that had this surgery, and learned from them how it all worked out for them. That is why I am sharing this with you.

How do I take my wrist to my chest when I don't even know that the seizure is happening? Well, this is how it is for me. You cannot wear the wristband when the magnet sticks to so many things around you—such as the dishwasher, the refrigerator, and the washing machine—so it was very hard to clean the house with it on my wrist. And these are just a few examples of how difficult it is wearing it.

On the day of the surgery, the neurosurgeon explained to me the consequences of having brain surgery on the right temporal lobe. I know I have all these in writing, but I am not doing this for myself. I am sharing this information in hopes that it will be of some help to you, to the doctors, or to someone you know. This epilepsy has made my life very difficult to live, and I don't believe people know about it. After reading this to my husband, he reminded me of a sentence I used to say in the first few years after meeting him continuously. He brought it up every once in a while with a smile on his face. He would put his hand in mine in the air and say, "You just don't understand."

For the second surgery, the doctors explained that I was going to have a loss of memory afterward. I said, "As long as I still know the people around, I am okay with it. But if that will happen, I don't want it. Okay, let's just get this done." I would do anything if there was a possibility that I would be seizure-free. This one was where they implanted a magnetic device in my chest, a vagus nerve stimulator (VNS).

I live in California; however, I have one of my medicines (an important one) flown in from New York. I hope to help you understand some of the questions about where you go and what to do with this condition.

By writing this book, who knows, maybe even some doctors and nurses may learn from this. I am hoping that it will inspire you or someone you know to look into all the options that are out there. I never thought I would be where I am today. I thought that epilepsy is a never-ending story. That is why I got to the point of not wanting to be in this world anymore. I would just have these questions in my mind: *Do I have to go through this again? Why? What did I do to deserve this?* I never know when I am going to have one or how strong and scary it is going to be. It is like being seen by your worst enemy, having no choice of where to go or what to do about it. Oh, and your insides are shaking at the same time. You have no control over anything—not inside or out.

I could go on and on to the point it's terribly frustrating when you have to deal with it. It all adds up to scary creatures that are irritating when I look back on how many times I have said the words *epilepsy* and *seizure*. I get excited when I talk to my friend in Georgia or anyone else in the first few minutes and ask, "Have you had any yet today? What was it like?"

I look at it this way. It was like the day my husband asked me to marry him. It was a life-changing experience that I would be happy about for the rest of my life. Now that I look back, the surgery is similar to a marriage. You need to get to know a person before you marry them. Just as I should have learned more about the effects of a surgery like this before jumping onto it. I do regret not looking into the outcome of all this. I could have investigated how other people with epilepsy were affected by this surgery. I was just too anxious to be seizure-free. I was willing to do anything to get rid of these scary déjà vu feelings that I was having day after day.

I remember when the doctor explained to me that they were going to insert a magnetic device into my chest, with wires connecting to my vagus nerve.

After this procedure, I have had a short-term memory problem. I also had a great many less seizures than I did before. They had me bring home a CPAP machine. I have not had any of those horrible petit mal seizures when I wake up. Those were the ones that upset me the most. I am so appreciative of this machine. I wear a mask every night when I go to sleep. Thankfully, it is very quiet and does not bother my husband's sleep at all. This has been a gigantic help to me not to wake up every morning with the same feeling I did after having those horrible seizures.

We just say our nightly prayers and give each other a quick good night kiss. Then (after he reminds me) I turn on my machine, and we both sleep well.

Now I don't know if I have already said this or not but who am I to complain? We can't have it all. That's not how it is in this life. So let's go back to the suicide attempts. I don't exactly remember what was going on that morning. I was just thinking, *Please, God, forgive me. I don't want to go through all this anymore.* Since I didn't know where to find a gun, I decided I would hang myself in the garage. I found a strong rope and tied it around some wood that was up above and stood on one of our tall dining room chairs. As I attempted to move the chair from under my feet, my husband's daughter came in to the garage and begged me to stop what I was doing. She had tears in her eyes, but I continued to try and move the chair with my feet. She quickly came toward me and held on to the chair, so I wasn't able to move it anymore.

She isn't a morning person. She doesn't get up early like I do. When I got the rope off that was around my neck and got off the chair, I apologized to her. People who don't have this problem have no idea how much it affects our daily lives. They don't understand all the disturbing feelings that it brings in our minds. Even some of the people that do have it might not understand the extent of it.

Every person is different. I have had a few seizures here there at church. This is one of the reasons my husband and I always sit in the front row. It is hard not to because after having one of my events, I have trouble walking between people to get away from it all and concentrate on how to deal with it. My husband always knows when I am having a seizure no matter what we are doing. I have total faith in him and that he will take care of me.

One of the medicines is known to bring on feelings of suicide, it is not for attention.

I feel 100 percent comfortable in the evenings and on the weekends. My husband and I spend a lot of time together.

From one epileptic to another, we may have a similar type of life, but every person is different. It is more about how we deal with what comes before us.

CHAPTER 8

A Little Humor

ONE DAY, WHEN my husband and I were in Los Angeles, California, coming back from one of my doctor's appointment, it was such a surprise to me when my husband and I were driving around the neighborhood that he knew pretty well. He asked me (out of the blue), "Do you want to get a tattoo?"

I surprisingly said, "Yeah, sure, why not?" What brought me to do this? I wasn't drunk; I had a clear mind. It came to the thoughts of putting something on me that relates to me, not with either of the words *epilepsy* or *seizure* but similar.

I looked at these tattoo designs and gave it a thought, *What kind of words or art will I like to have on my body for the rest of my life?*

For those of you who like tattoos, I am now with you. All my life, I had no desire to get one. I couldn't imagine having something on my body for the rest of my life. Well, not anything God did not created. What would I be proud of putting on my body and for others to see?

I am one of those people who change their mind frequently. That is why I am thankful that we have erasers and Wite-Out. Oh, and there is always that Delete button on our computers

I don't remember if before this day I had thought about what or where I would put this on me, but I came up with an idea of something I am going to deal with for the rest of my life. Then I felt comfortable with the choice of words that fit me just right. On my upper-right arm, what is it that fits me so perfectly? "Sorry, I don't remember."

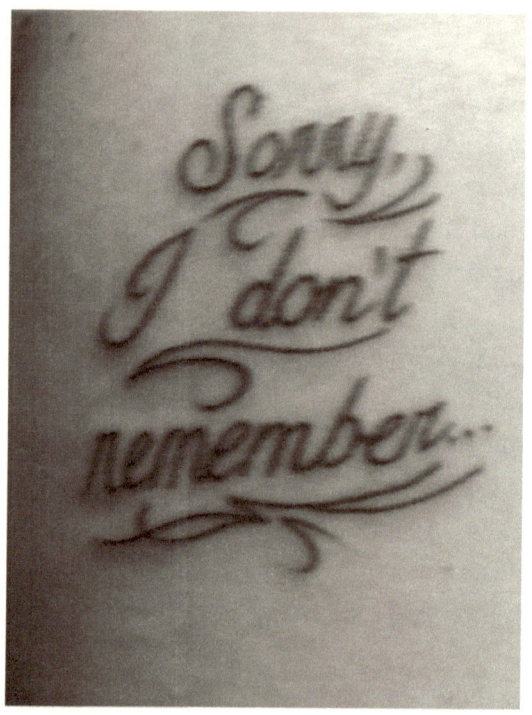

And since I got that, I was going to have to put this on my upper left arm, Oh yeah, "Please don't let me forget." That's kind of funny, huh? When I am wearing a short-sleeve top and I am discussing the trouble I have with my memory, I will definitely show them my two arms. I am sure it will bring a smile to their face. The one tattoo I have now does. So the smile will probably be bigger when I show them both of my arms.

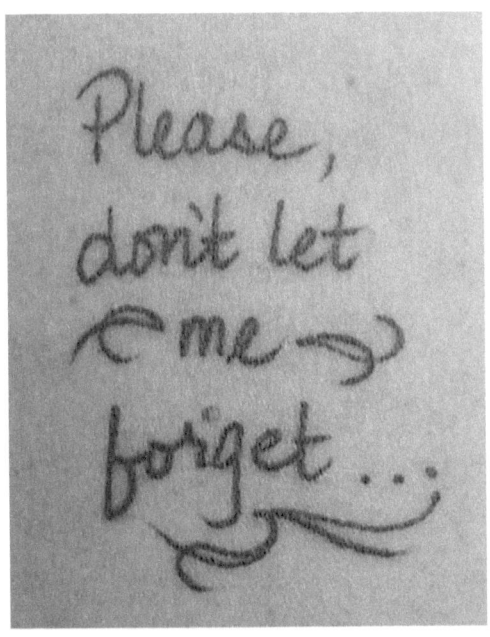

My husband picks me up from work, and he usually arrives before I get off work, waiting for me in the parking lot. He drives a big gray truck that he had for over a decade. Therefore, I know this truck pretty well. Yet one day, as I was waiting for him, I saw this truck that looked just like ours. Since I am always anxious to see him after work, I jumped into the truck. There was a man sitting in there alone. I didn't give it a second thought to look at this man. I just jumped in and put my purse on my lap. Less than a second later, I surprisingly said, "Sorry, wrong truck." The man smiled.

Something else that may bring a smile to your face or you may be able to relate to is when my girlfriend and I would go out dancing in different clubs and the lights were flashing on the dance floor. I had been told by my special friend that due to the lights, I often pass out and would have seizures. She would tell me that people thought I was drunk, but I don't even drink alcohol. The flashing lights could bring on my seizures.

CHAPTER 9

Through the Eyes of Loved Ones, Family, and Friends

David

I HAVE BEEN married to Stephanie, my lovely bride, for over fifteen years. During this time, it has involved a lot of changes.

In the beginning of our marriage, it was basically getting to know and learning how to deal with her seizures, coming to the understanding of the importance of patience and bringing me to a greater understanding of the extra time, care, and attention she requires.

In the early years of our marriage, her mom was very helpful in pointing a lot of these things out to me, certain things that I had never realized. Another life-changing event in our marriage was after the surgical removal of a part of her brain on the right temporal lobe. The surgery affected a part of her memory, bringing on a whole other set of challenges. I had never understood how important, how big a part of our lives a memory plays. Things like scheduling her rides to get to work or remembering to take her meds or even what day of the week it is.

All these are things that a person without her disability takes for granted.

Stephanie can meet someone and not remember them five minutes later. It all affects her self-confidence, insecurities, frustrations, fears, and sense of loneliness.

I believe our greatest rewards come from helping others, putting ourselves in other people's shoes. Although it isn't always easy loving and being married to Steph, it has been the greatest blessing from God above, and I wouldn't change it for the world.

Adriana

Stephanie and I met in school. We both screwed up in high school and needed to get back to getting our lives together, and from the day we met, we were inseparable. We started to learn about each other. She had explained that she was in a car accident that left her with epilepsy and a slight short-term memory problem. I started to do research on my own to better understand what Stephanie was going through and how I could best help her. I had never met anyone with epilepsy, so I had no clue what to do.

Over the years, I learned how to deal with each one of the different types of seizures Stephanie would have. I would never fully understand what Steph went through. I would have to have a seizure myself to fully understand, which I knew Stephanie would never even wish on her worst enemy.

We would be at a nightclub, dancing, and she would end up having a seizure. We'd be thrown out because they thought she was too drunk to be there. Other times, people thought she was crazy and would yell mean things at her. Half the time, people will try to call 911, and I would have to explain to them that she has epilepsy and ask them to please not do that as I will help her.

There are many other examples of the things that she had to go through. Being her best friend, I viewed her seizures from the outside. She had different types of seizure. She had the small déjà vu ones, where she would look far off and be almost dazed and confused. Another one was when her eyes started to twitch and get really big in her face and her lips would twitch to the side, and then as soon as it started, her hand would start scratching her thigh. For being somebody who didn't have epilepsy or seizures, it was very scary to see someone go through something like that. I would talk her through them to try to keep her calm because the seizure would scare her—actually, I should say terrify her!

For the big grand mal ones, I would have to get down on the floor and put her head between my thighs so her head would bounce off each thigh and never ever put anything in her mouth and just wait until it was over.

Throughout the years, Stephanie has had different surgeries to help improve her quality of life with epilepsy and essentially try to cure it. With each surgery or procedure came a new set of troubles. This last one had caused Steph's memory to get worse. I couldn't even count how many times I prayed that these things would be taken away. I know God has his own timing and he is working on her. I have no doubt.

Over all these years, Stephanie has taught me courage and strength through all obstacles. She has taught me to lean on God and lean not on my own understanding. She is my best friend until the end!

Debbie

Stephanie is my sister's only child. When she was born, I could not spend enough time with her. I watched her whenever I could. I adored my little niece, she even lived with me for a few years. When she got into her car accident and had her brain injury, I went to see her in the hospital. She remembered me, but she didn't remember my son or even that she had a son. There were many struggles that came along because of her brain injury and because of her memory loss. She had a very hard time accepting that she couldn't drive with them.

They tried to figure out what was causing the seizures, then what part of the brain they were from. Then they found out they were from two parts of the brain. Stephanie had been through so many struggles since her accident. Different smells would bring on her seizures. She would wake up with these horrible feelings or auras. She would be terrified. It had been very difficult for her and everyone around her.

Through all her struggles, she went to college and worked several jobs over the years until she found the perfect job for her. Steph has been at her present employer for over ten years. She met and married her husband, who is perfect for her. They are partners in life. When she told me about this project of writing a book, I told her I would be happy to help her in any way I could to get what she had to say about her life and what she'd been through and to get that out to people whom it could help.

Stephanie is an amazing inspiration to those with or without disabilities. She has taught me to take each day, one day at a time. I love you.

Aunt Debbie

CHAPTER 10

Unconditional Love

OVER TIME, AS I have had these seizures, there is no way I would be where I am today if I didn't have the love, care, and support that the people who are around me have generously provided. I also appreciate the intelligent doctors and the hospital that I am associated with now. The hospital gave me a chance and made a huge difference in my life.

The man of my dreams and I have been married fifteen years now. Our relationship is definitely what you would call unconditional love. He has seen my seizures at their worst, even before we got married. I recently found out that he went to a bookstore when we were dating to find out everything he could about epilepsy.

I am happy with the thoughts of my mother and others who knew I was in good hands, with my husband taking care of me for the rest of my life, before they died.

CHAPTER 11

Where I Am Now

IF YOU ARE still suffering with epilepsy and are having trouble with it, don't lose hope. Just look around. That is what I did. God directed me to the right place at the right time. It made a tremendous difference in my life. If I didn't follow where he directed me, I wouldn't be where I am today.

I don't know. Maybe this will inspire other people to tell their story about the disability they have and all the pain and suffering that they go through. We need to stick together and let people know about our troubles so that we can get through all these—not alone but together. The more people know, the less difficult it may be.

I don't think we talk about our feelings enough. How is someone going to care if we don't share? This may have something to do with us being afraid of how others will judge us. All our situations are different, but in some way or another, someone out there will just listen to what it is we are going through. Many of us need to vent. I know I do because it is a weight off my back when I do. God gave us these incredible minds, voices to speak, and hands to write, so let's use them. Our God wants us to work together to make this life easier to live in because we all know that it is not easy for anyone.

I just need to go with the flow and live in the moment. I have always admired people who are able to do this. I just need to get in the habit of it. My everyday challenges would be a lot less stressful for me if I do. Sounds good, huh? It would be a great weight off my back. I am sure people around me would like it if I did this. So now that I am giving this a thought, I would like to start this today. I can do this!

It is amazing and upsetting that our brain can see visions of things that we have seen before but have never happened. They are similar to dreams that you have had. These are the petit mal seizures, also known as déjà vu seizures. You are in a totally different world when this is happening. You have no care of what is going on around you. You can have a gun pointed to your head, and instead of worrying about that, you are more interested in the visions that you are seeing in your mind. Why can't I just tell these sights to leave me alone, then I would be able to go on doing what I am doing? But it's just not like that. They have full control over your mind. I am curious are there people out there who are able to tell the seizure to just leave them alone and overcome them with no trouble?

The feelings are so disturbing.

It is so annoying to me that bright lights, smells, and tastes of food can trigger these feelings. When I say feelings, I am referring to the petit mal seizures that are not as noticeable. These seizures are not as common as the grand mal; however, I feel that they are more annoying than the other ones. When the episode stops, I don't know that it has happened. I am just exhausted. Afterward, I usually fall asleep no matter where I am, and sometimes when I wake up, I ask them why am I so tired.

They will say, "You just had a seizure."

I just reply, "Okay, that makes sense." Now when I have a grand mal, it is different. These don't seem to be as bad to me as the other ones. With these, I don't get those terrible feelings. I have been told that I just fall down, pass out, and shake around a little bit. I don't get as tired after these.

And even if they only last a few seconds or a minute, they are tremendously scary. Sometimes, the ones that last just a few seconds are more intense than the other ones, especially when my insides are shaking and I had absolutely no control of what is going on.

CHAPTER 12

Troubling Relationships

MY RELATIONSHIP WITH my son has been troublesome over the years. He was seven months old when we were in the car accident. When I came out of the coma, I was told that my son survived. I don't remember the details of this day; however, I do remember asking, "What son?" My mother then explained to me what I was doing in the hospital and that my son will be all right. He had no injuries. I recognized her but not my son. This was a life-changing experience.

As he was growing up, he was so close to my mother. She cared for my son as if he were hers. I ask myself, why does she get to be the mother of my son? This made me jealous of their relationship. It was difficult for me to watch her care for my son the way I wanted to. She was able to get him things that he wanted and needed, whereas I was not. I was jealous of their relationship. She gave both of us all her attention. I would say she gave him a little bit more. Yet that was understandable, being that he was a child and I was an adult. I was eighteen when I gave birth to my son, so some would say I was a young adult who was not ready to be a mother. Now when I look back, I totally agree with that.

Yet I couldn't do it without her and all she did for him. I wasn't just jealous; I was envious of everyone who was in good health. As we all know, people may look like they are in good health but are not. I know

I am one of those people. This is why we should not judge a book by its cover. We just need to keep our eyes and ears open so that we can help one another in any way we can. It was really me being angry about my situation. I was always looking into the moment, not the surrounding circumstances. The stress about all this brought on more and more seizures.

I have already seen a huge change in my life. I don't know you, but if you know change is positive, don't give up. Look into whatever you can for some kind of change. We only live once on earth, and we need to give it our all to enjoy the place.

Well, it was Mother's Day, and I luckily came up with an idea of what I was going to do for my mother on this day. Instead of buying her a present she might like, knowing that she loves to watch movies, I asked her if she would like to go to the movies, my treat. This was the perfect date for us because we always had the TV on watching movies.

My husband David, would often ask me, "How do you remember the last one?" And what he was referring to were the scriptures in the Bible that were always helpful to me. I would memorize one of them. I usually needed him to remind me of the first couple of words that I could not remember. Then I remembered it.

Our memory is on the right side of our brain. What happened to my memories was a result of the surgery on my right temporal lobe. Fortunately, I do not have a choice to choose what I want to remember and what I don't want to remember. I just need to have faith, which is important. And because I cannot do anything, I sometimes feel like I have the mind of a child, but now is the time to grow up and accept this.

I am pleased with the changes in my attitude and the lessons I have learned. As I have said before, the past is the past. Let's just forget about it and move on.

Everyone around me has done their best in caring for me through all the hardships that come with this disorder, but nobody knows all about the experience themselves. The more we learn from one another, the better. This is extremely important to all of us.

Just think positive and keep your eyes and ears and mind open to the thought that there is someone out there somewhere who will care and listen to your feelings about what is going on in your mind and body.

We often look at the negative things in life before we look at the positive ones. I know I do. *There is always that one or more person who are stronger than you.*

This may come to their mind and definitely comes to my mind. I couldn't imagine losing my arm or my leg. We need to stop being selfish and jealous of people that have more than we do.

It is similar to an earthquake. You have no idea when they're coming or going or what the outcome may actually be. I recently used the computer to look and see how it was working for others. I found it to be helpful.

This book is a learning tool for people who have a disability, especially epilepsy. It is a self-help book to give you ideas and thoughts and the determination that there may be a solution to the difficulties with your disability. It is difficult for us to live with epilepsy. Some people, more than others, I am one of them, had an extremely hard time dealing with this condition. I am here for you to relate to all the life experiences, the good and the bad, that has brought me from where I once was to where I am today.

I know many other people with medical conditions that are much worse; however, this is not a competition of who is going or dealing with more than the other. Both of you can understand that it is worse than it looks. Nobody, even the person who have seizures, can understand the irritation that we have to deal with. The physical part of this isn't as bad as the mental irritation that we have to deal with.

I know I've seen this before. What is going to happen next? You don't think about your body shaking, you drooling, or you urinating in your pants. All you care about is that this is happening. You usually don't know what you are doing during all this. All you care about is to make this feeling stop.

I'm sure there are many people in this world who just want their life over with. Some of us are stronger than others. Here's another example of the trouble I had with my family, my husband, and my son, who was with us for a few days. Since he was leaving this morning and I had something I needed to get from the store, I asked him if he could drop me off. I'm sure most of you can relate to something like this happening to you every once in a while, but how would you feel about having an occurrence like this every day? It is difficult not being able to drive. I just got done watching a show on television, and I don't remember if she is just like me and just wanted to end it all. Yes, God must have felt it was not our time to leave this life. If she could get this off her mind, then why can't I? We need to open our eyes and minds to see what is out there for us to have a better life.

I hope that through my story, you have a better idea that everyone has some kind of problem and sometimes it might be a great many difficulties. But this epilepsy has definitely been the worst. The best advice I can give you is to live every day as if it were your last. I personally have a very hard time, and I am ready to go. But obviously, people around me disagree. I need to remember this because I myself have always had a problem all my life. Epilepsy has made me more miserable. People have no idea. I have a lot of families and friends. I am just a good actress, just trying to get through all these obstacles in my everyday life. I love my husband. But as I say You Need To Love Yourself, I just need to repeat to myself the scripture Psalm 37:7, "Rest in the Lord and wait patiently for Him."

And even if it only lasts for a few seconds or a minute, they're tremendously scary, especially when my insides are shaking and I have absolutely no control of anything that is going on. Sometimes, when I am having a seizure, I care more about the visions I am seeing than anything that is happening around me, even how intense the shaking is. If there was a gun in front of me, I would ask the person to shoot me so that this never happens again.

We all need to wake up with this thought: *What can we do to make my life better?* But in the past, I would go to sleep hoping that I would not wake up again. For many years, I would continuously wake up in the morning with the same feeling that I had while I was having a petit mal seizure. I am sure I had brought this to the attention of the first hospital that I went to for years. My family and I had no idea what was causing this to happen. I don't even know if this hospital did. Then I went to UCLA. They discovered that it was happening because I was not getting enough oxygen to my brain in my sleep. I was having petit mal seizures in my sleep. I was surprised that this was happening. What would bring these on in my sleep? Therefore, they introduced me to the CPAP machine. Since I had been using the machine, I have had no trouble with waking up miserably, like I did before. This has been a tremendous help in my life.

I and others around me have noticed a positive difference in my attitude about life. There is now a reason to live. I feel that it's possible that I will be seizure-free in the future. Whereas before, I had no idea that I would be this close to possibly getting over the troubles that I have suffered for over twenty years.

Now I feel that there is an opportunity to enjoy this life. I still have a difficult time with my memory, and I always will. But that doesn't bother me compared to epilepsy. I can deal with having a really bad memory. And if I were to have a grand mal seizure once in a great while, I can deal with that too. I don't want to, of course, but that is nothing compared to where I once was.

I now feel that I am supposed to be here on this earth for a reason. It has been quite a challenge to get me to where I am today. And I am thankful to God for guiding me through all that I have done. And most of all, I thank him for bringing me together with the right people in my life.

Before my accident, I might have heard someone say the words *epilepsy* or *seizure* once or twice. Yet I had no idea what exactly what they were talking about. There must not have been any details about what it was all about. This is why I am writing this book. I want to help you and others to get an idea of what comes with this disorder, especially for those of you who are new to all this.

I just wish I could see what it is like when I have a seizure. I don't remember if I have ever seen anyone have a seizure in person.

Many people have told me that my eyes roll back, shake a little, and fall down. I am not as tired after having one of these, as opposed to having a petit mal seizure. I can, after a couple of minutes, usually go back to doing whatever it was I was doing before the seizure occurred. These do not bother me half as much as the scary petit mal seizures.

One day, not long ago, I was staying the night at my best friend's house, and we used the computer together and found a site where it showed people having seizures. This was very interesting to me. As we were watching it, she shared with me which ones were similar to the ones that I have. This meant so much to me. I also wish I could see what it was like when the doctors did the three surgeries, but oh well. It is too late now. I don't believe I will be having another surgery, but if you will be having one, keep all this in mind. You, too, may be curious of these things.

I just remember the neurosurgeon explaining to me on the day of the surgery (on my right temporal lobe) that my memory was going to be affected by this. This is because it was where the doctor was going to take a piece out of my brain (about the size of a quarter). I definitely remember the doctor asking me, "You are going to have short-term memory loss for the rest of your life. Is that all right?"

I then, without a second thought, replied, "Sure, as long as I know who the people in my life are." Almost everybody has some trouble with their memory as they age. It will just happen to me sooner. Plus, I was already impaired from the car accident when I was eighteen years old. Since I am forty-three years old now, I would do it. I am a person who is known to change their mind a lot but not about this. I was ready when the doctor was ready. The sooner, the better. I was in great need of any change in my life, and I have total faith that UCLA doctors know what they are doing.

And the doctors were right when they said "short-term memory loss." I remembered who everyone was after the surgery, and they were also right when they said that I was going to have "short-term memory loss." Here are a few examples of the daily troubles that I have with this:

1. Did I take my medication?

2. Do I work today?
3. Did I schedule my transportation to get to work?
4. Did I brush my teeth and wash my hair?
5. Did I feed the dogs?
6. Where did I put my keys and my phone?

I am sure that you all can relate to these kinds of questions. You probably ask yourselves the same thing; however, these are just a couple that come to my mind more than once. After I try to answer them, I ask them to myself again and again. It gets really annoying. This happens every day throughout the day, not just every now and then.

I don't have the attention span of those around me, so it is often that I have a hard time holding conversations with people that I do not know very well and people that do not know my situation. I do the best I can with what I got.

This is just a simple book for those who can understand and care and maybe relate to a disability and all its difficulties. I guess this is what you would call an autobiography, yet I am not writing this for myself. This is for you or someone you know who wants to know some differences with epilepsy. I am definitely not a writer. I don't even read books. I am talking with you about one of the troubles that you might be able to relate so you might be able to change. Even if you haven't had surgery, you could be going through the same problem I have. I have terrible trouble, as the surgeon explained to me before the surgery.

I would often find myself upstairs at work with a cup of water in my hand. I would not know what was going on in the beginning. I would ask whoever was close to me as to why I was there. Then as they were explaining what had happened so quick, that would come to mind. So I would realize I was not on my ten-minute break. So yes, it was another seizure.

Having Another Brain Surgery

Next month, I will be having another surgery. This will be on my left temple. they took something out. Now they want to put something on the left side—an RNS. I recently spoke to a person who had this procedure done a year ago, and they said it had been successful for them. My doctor shared with me that it will also be an improvement to my situation. Surgeons jumped at this opportunity and brought it to my attention. I was extremely excited to give it a try. I was told before by people in my life that I might not remember, but they understand me. I wasn't going to let anything get in the way of having the surgery. I am disabled, and I am still determined to get these out of my life.

I look back at the VNS surgery. I am writing this book to let you know that there is hope. If you haven't found the right doctors or medicines, that's all right. You just haven't found it yet. Let's keep our eyes open to what is out there. Don't give up.

I do not like talking about myself more than the average person, but I am thankful for the people around me who understand this. Of course, I would like to talk more about the world, such as who was in the movie. To them, I just need to ask. It is disturbing that I have a hard time keeping up with all the people whose opinion matters and who understand and is able to overlook it.

I am so grateful to God for the day he brought to my mind that I could continue with his disability. With the way it was, there had to be some kind of change—a big change. For over a decade of these continuous seizures that I was having, almost every day, I was miserable. I just want to die, and I have no fear of death, especially when I'm being tortured. I gave it some thought and asked myself, What can I do? There has to be some kind of change.

Share with others. If we don't share our experience, then people will have no idea what we're going through. You might just say "I had a seizure." There is so much more to it than that. We need to let them know everything about it in detail; however, I know from experience that some of the ones I've had, I don't even remember the time. I have no idea what's happening, and somebody else makes it scary for us. I will give you an idea of what I'm talking about in another chapter.

Sometimes I get a warning sign that it is about to happen. This will be for a couple of seconds before it turns into controlling me. I sometimes don't have the warning that it is about to happen. These seizures have total control of my actions. I am no longer a slave to fear. I am a child of God. I stand in the hope of a new life that I want. I am alive, and I wait patiently for him (Psalm 37:7). We're able to be filled with the Holy Spirit. Live every day. I am a patient person.

This is something I will never forget. It wasn't just from drugs; I was anorexic too. The love of my life at that time told me I was fat and ugly, so this told me that I was not the only one who had childish behavior.

Here is where I am right now as I am sharing all my life. Earlier this morning, I was told by my husband I hit the footboard while having a seizure. I woke up today with no idea of what had happened. I asked myself what happened and why my chin was swollen with dried blood all over. It is irritating when you wake up having no idea of what happened just a few hours before. My mind was totally blank.

In the past, I would have some idea. Ever since I had short-term memory problem, this had been a great surprise to me as it would be for you. Some of you might be surprised, and some of you might just blow it off and move on with things right away. I wish I could do that. I am sick and tired of these seizures having so much control of my life. Babe, on my mind, I would always ask, When am I going to have another one? What is going to happen? When I do, my next thought is, Is there anything I can do to get them to stop? I have tried so much—three surgeries and medications from New York. What now? I am sure that some people would have said to not let it get the best of you. You have so much in your life to appreciate. God won't give you anything you can't handle. To tell you the truth, I do not want to handle this anymore. I want to just give up.

I have no doubt in my mind that he doesn't love me because of how I look. It is because of who I am. He knows me inside and out. Also, because of my love for him and the Lord God. It is such a nice feeling to be totally in love with your mate even after fifteen years of marriage. There is more and more love every day.

If you haven't found this type of person in your life yet, don't give up. They are out there somewhere. Don't worry about this epilepsy problem that we have. The right person for you will accept you just the way you are. They will have faith in you, that you, too, may be seizure-free one day. You need your mate and just need to work on this problem together, just as my husband and I have.

Our Pets, Our Heroes

My husband and I have two dogs. One is a large golden retriever, which my husband claims is his dog, and the other is a smaller one, which my husband says is mine. They are buddies. They get along just right. They are both very special to me.

My husband works very hard, and he needs to take a nap every once in a while. And both of the dogs know that if he is home in the middle of the day and the bedroom door is closed, they don't go there! They are both pretty good about that.

My husband was working the night shift this week, so hours ago, he was in the bedroom, sleeping. My small dog was lying in front of our bedroom door. I knew he wanted to be in the room with my husband, yet if I let him in, he would probably wake my husband up. I didn't get up. I continued to lie on the couch and tried to ignore it. The next thing I knew, my husband was next to me. He put me on the couch and explained to me what had happened. He said that my dog just woke him up. He was scratching at the door and barking up a storm. He said that he was a little irritated about the dog waking him up but that he got over it when he found me lying on the living room floor. If my husband didn't pick me up and put me on the couch, I probably would have just wondered why I was on the floor. Things like this have happened a great many times over the years. I would ask myself and others, "Where am I? Why am I here?" This was after I had a seizure that I didn't know happened, whereas some of them, I had an idea that it occurred.

I will tell you another good example of this in a minute. Let's just think, What if I had hit my head on the coffee table or something like that and had another brain injury and my husband didn't wake up for hours? I am so thankful for the loving and caring dogs I have.

Another time I had a scary moment was when I had a seizure while I was cooking. I had a horrible experience with a seizure where I burned eight of my ten fingers. At the time, my husband rushed me to the burn center of the hospital. I had no idea of what happened. I only remember sticking my hands out the window of his truck, questioning what had happened to have me in this excruciating pain. As he was driving, he explained to me that my third-degree burns on my two hands were due to me putting both of my hands in a pot of boiling hot water, as I was cooking him dinner. He was in the shower when I did this, so he had no idea that it had happened until his sister told him about it.

My husband, after a long day's work, would enjoy the taste of cheese. He loves mac and cheese, so before he jumped in the shower, I offered to make him some. Since that was the only food I cook on the stove it was no problem. Well I don't know maybe the dogs were barking when this happened too. Something got my sister-in-law's attention to come into the room. She was in the next room when I did it, and she must have heard something. I was told that she tried to take the pot away from me as I had placed it on my left cheek. I thank the Lord that she found me as I was doing this. If she hadn't, who knows what could have happened. I might have been about to pour the water on my face. Luckily, I didn't. It just left an open spot on my face, which healed just right.

I didn't understand why the doctors were cutting skin off my legs. It was to put over the third-degree burns on my eight burned fingers. What caused these burns? I don't remember anything about this.

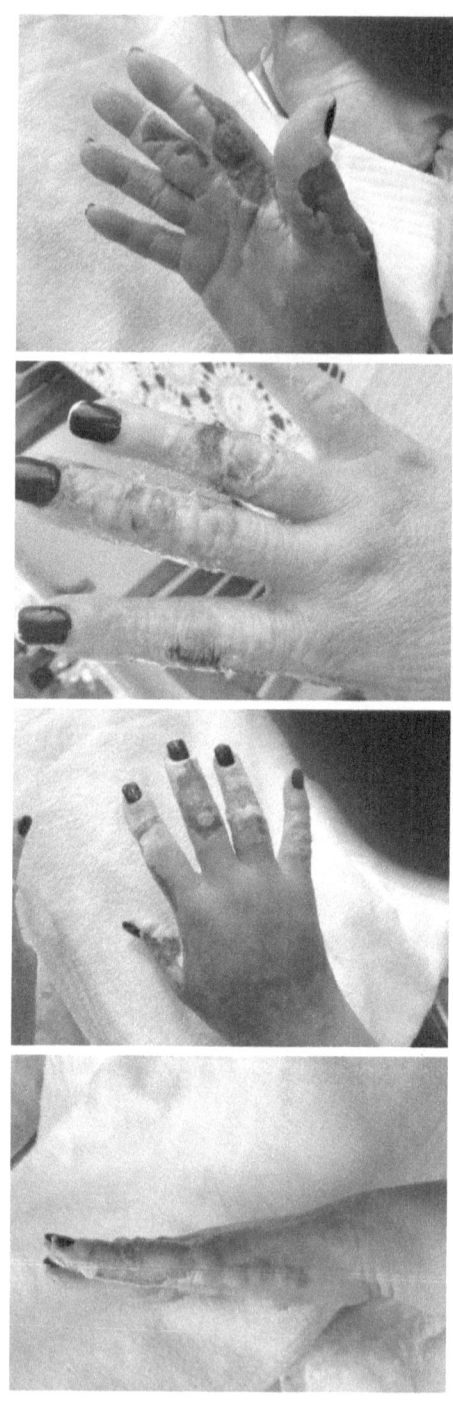

When I came around from all the strong meds I was in the hospital, my husband was by my side, explaining to me that I was making his macaroni and cheese. I had one of my regular petit mal seizures. During my seizure, I picked up the pan of boiling water that was on the stove and put it up to my face. Who knows what could have happened next. It left spots on my face, but this burn wasn't even half as bad as the burns on my fingers. Think about all we do with our hands. Well, I couldn't do much for quite a while.

Have you ever had this kind of problem with your memory? I'm not talking about every once in a while; I'm talking about daily. Here are some of the annoyances that I deal with almost every day. Everyone has, at some point, some hard time remembering something. I am a forty-three year-old who has the memory of an eighty-year-old person. Let me share with you what it is like for a person who has had a portion about the size of a quarter taken out of their brain. It was when I had the surgery on my right temporal lobe. The doctors had explained to me that I was going to have a hard time remembering. I never assumed it was going to be difficult.

Here are some examples of how it is at work. I had a hard time remembering one of my customers on Monday afternoon at the grocery store. I was bagging items. I saw a man who looked familiar to me. As I was bagging his items, I looked at him and questioned where I knew him from. This happened an awful lot. I was pretty sure he saw the questionable look on my face and explained that he was the pastor of the church I attended the day before. With a heartfelt smile on his face and being a pastor, I knew he wasn't offended by this. Of course, he wasn't surprised. He knew about the surgery and what the consequences were going to be. But isn't that funny? I'd been watching him preach for years, but I didn't recognize him.

I was at work one day when a woman asked me if I needed a ride home from work. My home was the only one exit off the freeway from the store where I work. I said *sure* since it was going to be a while until my husband was going to be able to pick me up. I don't know how this happened since my house was just up the hill, but as she was driving toward my house, I somehow got her and I lost. Boy, did I feel bad about this.

My mother was overweight when I was growing but not my dad. Her being a great cook that she was might have had something to do with it. She didn't drink alcohol, just a lot of coffee. Anyways, it probably had something to do with me wanting to be skinny.

In high school, I hung out with people that were older than me and had already had drugs in their life. So it was easy for me to get them. Marijuana was one of the most common. That was where most people started out. That wasn't the one for me because, as many of you might know, that was the one that makes you hungry after smoking it. I discovered meth, and with that drug, you are never hungry. You may go many days and not desire food. I still, to this day, don't like the taste of alcohol. Thank goodness. But meth, known as speed at times, was hard for me to deal with because it was the one you couldn't get enough of. The more I did, the skinnier I became.

I will always remember my mother telling me that when I got in this particular accident, I only weighed eighty-nine pounds. I was skin and bones. My sons father would tell me I was fat. He made me feel ugly.

Well, I still had a problem with my weight. I had about thirty pounds to lose. I did a lot of walking, and I went to the gym when I got the chance. I was just thankful my husband would stay with me no matter my weight. If I was given a choice of winning the lottery or being seizure-free for the rest of my life, without a second thought, I would choose to be seizure-free not only for myself but for the many people around me. It would be another wonderful gift from God.

No worries, we can get through this together—one epileptic to another. We may have a similar type of life, but every person is different. It is more about how we deal with what comes before us.

It was 6:45 a.m., and I woke up about fifteen minutes ago. I just looked in my medicine container, and there were no meds in the Sunday-morning spot. Being almost positive that I haven't take them yet, I got discouraged about what to do. The afternoon ones and the evening ones were there, but what happened to the morning ones? Well, no matter what happened to them, I had to have some meds in my body or I might have a seizure. We don't want that to happen, do we? So I just gave up on guessing what had already happened, and took Monday-morning's instead. Hopefully, everything will be all right.

Next month, I will be having another brain surgery. This will be on my left temporal lobe. I will be having an RNS implanted in my brain.

I recently spoke to a person who had this procedure done a year ago, and they said it has been successful for them. My doctor shared with me that it will also be an end to my situation. The surgeon brought this opportunity to my attention. I was extremely excited to give it a try, just as I was with the other surgeries. I was told before that I would probably have more trouble with my short-term memory, which I have now found to be true. Luckily, I know who the important people in my life are. I might not remember what we talked about just a few hours ago, but they have been very helpful, caring, and understanding about reminding me of what is going on around me.

I was supposedly born with epilepsy. This was what my main doctor told my husband. She said that the car accident activated it. Or was the accident brought on by my first seizure?

There are many ways to look at this. What comes to my mind is, Would I have been born with this condition and suffered my entire childhood with it? I would definitely be a totally different person. Maybe they wouldn't have bothered me as much as they do now.

Maybe God felt this is the time?

The feelings are so disturbing that I just want to give you an idea of how extreme and scary these feelings are.

Well, I want you all to remember that the past is the past. So let go of the past and let's concentrate on what's going on now. Yet I do have some more to explain about where I was then to where I am today, so please bear with me.

He is the best author of all times. As we all know, he didn't write the book yet. I do believe he had a lot to do with it. He guided the right people to share his Word, bringing it all into perspective that we can be good people with whatever we are going through in our hard time on this earth.

Since I was anxious about the thought of having no more of these stupid seizures, I said, "Don't worry about that. I am ready to do this, whatever the consequences might be." I wasn't thinking about the future. I was only thinking of the possibility of being seizure-free.

Over the last week, I have been looking all over my house and threw away papers and even my husband's. Where are they? Did I or someone else throw them away? These are the first chapters of this book. I felt totally comfortable about how I had written them, but of course, I have rough drafts. So I will start over, but it won't be exactly how I wrote it before.

I have a habit of hiding things that are important to me.

What would you do?

So why am I so affected by my lack of memory? I have an easier time with that, then the seizures occurring spontaneously.

When I have a seizure, if I am standing still or in a chair, all I need is for someone to speak to me to distract me from the visions. Do not touch me. I am unaware of anything going on around me when I am having a seizure. I am concentrating on the visions in my mind. This is true when I am having a petit mal (déjà vu) seizure. If I am having a grand mal (tonic-clonic seizure) seizure, unless I am bleeding from my occasional falling down, you do not need to call for emergency services or 911.

Let's Give It a Try

God will take care of us. We just need to give him the chance. And the best way of doing that is having a relationship with him and pray about all that we deal with. It sure has been some help to me.

Many years ago, I looked into starting a support group for those of us who suffer from epilepsy. We could relate to one another and learn from each other's experiences. I had it all planned out. I was so excited about it. It was for family and friends too.

I don't remember how I found the people with epilepsy. I was just hoping that it would be successful. It didn't go on for a very long. A few people showed up, but overtime it was difficult for all of us to get to the same place at the same time. Well, I tried. I may try again in the future.

Since day 1, I have had a horrible time remembering to take my medication. My mother would ask me here and there, but in those days, I didn't take it as seriously as I do now. This is probably why I was having one seizure after another. For years, I was waking up almost every morning having a seizure. The first hospital I went to over a decade ago never looked into why this was happening. Luckily, the one that I go to now found out right away that it was happening because I was having the seizures in my sleep. That made total sense to me. After so many years, why didn't I think of that? I was going to sleep hoping I would not wake up. This is just one of the reasons why I attempted suicide. I have learned from many of the people around me that "God will not give us more than we can handle."

Until I met my husband, I had never heard these words or any scriptures at all. I had memorized a few, but not as many as I would like to. I couldn't even memorize my husband's phone number. Thank goodness for cell phones.

The doctor said that I was going to have a bad memory before I had the surgery, but I would have let them cut off my right arm if they needed to. I am right-handed. That was how intense the seizures were.

Sure, the doctors know where they come from and what to do about getting rid of them, but they don't know the intense feelings that come with them. Patients can explain it to them, but there is so much more to it than words can say.

I think of it like this. I am sure that there is a lot more to cancer, AIDS, and other diseases. As I have been told and understood, nobody in this world has the exact same thing or feelings about anything. God made us all different.

They Make Me Feel

I don't know about you, but for me, the negative thoughts overpower the positive ones. In the past, I would lie down to sleep hoping I would not wake up. That was what it was like when I was having the morning petit mal seizures daily. Do you ever feel tortured by all this that you have to deal with, asking others, even God, "What did I do to deserve this? Is this ever going to end?" There I go again, thinking negative. I know many people have worse medical troubles, but this is not a competition. I just want you to know that this is what it is like in the life of someone with epilepsy. We are all different. I still have the grand mal seizures. But I don't know when I have them, so it is not as upsetting to me.

CHAPTER 13

Don't Lose Hope

FOR OVER A decade, I was going to a low-income hospital that took our Medi-cal, and all they did was change the dosage of my medication that I was taking. They never talked about any types of surgery.

One day God brought to my attention that I needed to look into finding more help. This was when I was on the verge of suicide. I needed to find a hospital that could give me a higher level of care, specifically for my needs. Finally, out of the blue, the thought of looking into finding the right hospital for me came to mind. It was one that I had only heard great things about. I was inspired to look into it. I didn't want to give up.

I planned on getting there on my own. In a car, it took over an hour or two to get there from where I lived at the time. I didn't tell anyone about this adventure. I figured out the bus schedule, and I needed to take five busses to get there. This was the first time I had ridden on a city bus.

Luckily, the hospital took me in with the insurance I had. It was known as Medi-cal. It was the type of insurance for people like me on government assistance. God was with me every step of the way.

CHAPTER 14

A Huge Help

FOR OVER TWENTY years, I woke up almost every morning having scary feelings. They were the same feelings I had many times after having a seizure. I shared all this with the doctors and nurses at the first hospital I stayed at, but they never did anything to investigate why I was having these morning seizures. When I say morning seizures, I meant that I was having them every morning when I wake up. This went on for many years.

So one day, I said to myself, "I can't go on with living this way. There has got to be a solution to this, or else, I am going to give up." That was how upsetting these seizures were. And these were the petit mal seizures that I was talking about. If they were grand mal ones, the ones I wouldn't know I had, I just don't remember when I have them now. Therefore, I went to a new, well-known, competent hospital. They gave me a few tests and found out what it was all about. After one of my overnight stays at the hospital, I found out from the neurologist that I was having seizures in my sleep. Why did it take so long to figure this out? Why didn't I figure this out? The doctor explained to me that I wasn't getting enough oxygen to my brain during my sleep. Before I was introduced to the CPAP machine, I would wake up almost every morning with scary and nervous feelings. I would start the day irritated by these feelings. What is this all about? I would ask myself. Did I have a bad dream? I don't know why I didn't look into this for so many years.

For all the years that I was going to that county hospital, they never said anything about this.

After going to UCLA (the best hospital around), they assured me that they would find out what was bringing these morning feelings up. No, it was not a bad dream; it was about me having seizures in my sleep.

Another huge help to me was when one of my doctors informed me of a special medication for epilepsy that just came out and advised me to look into it. They had it in two other states but not in California. She gave my husband and me all the information that we needed to be able to get it.

CHAPTER 15

Scriptures

HERE ARE A few scriptures that you might want to keep, especially when you are depressed about anything:

Cast your cares on the Lord and He will sustain you; he will never let the righteous fall. (Psalm 55: 22)

Today is the day the Lord has made, let us rejoice and be glad in it. (Psalms 118:24)

Do not be anxious about anything, but in every situation, by prayer and petition, with thanksgiving, present your requests to God. (Philippians 4:6 NIV)

The eyes of the Lord are on the righteous and his ears are attentive to their cry. (Psalm 34: 15)

Come close to God, God will come close to you. (James 4:8)

Rest in the Lord, and wait patiently for him. (Psalm 37:7)

I am no longer a slave to fear, I am a child of God. (Philippians 4:6)

The eyes of the Lord are on the righteous and his ears are attentive. (Psalm 34:15)

A FINAL THOUGHT

I AM WRITING this book in hopes that it will be of some help to you and others. Who knows, maybe some doctors and nurses may learn from this. All of us with epilepsy need to stick together because only us with seizures know what it is truly all about.

I tried to start a support group years ago, but it was difficult for us to all get together on the same day at the same time. We were all dependent on others and their busy schedule. Why do I care so much about not being able to drive? My grandmother lived until she was eighty-nine, and she never drove a car. If she could do it, so could I.

One day I went in to a bookstore, and I looked for a book about a person who suffers with epilepsy. There was nothing like it. Well, not that I could remember anyways. God definitely brought this book ideas to my attention. I just hope that some of you can relate or just learn from my experiences with this disease.

www.ingramcontent.com/pod-product-compliance
Lightning Source LLC
Chambersburg PA
CBHW031536210526
45464CB00003B/1036